Preparing For a Fast

Preparing For a Fast

Fasting

Rev. Carolyn Young Davis

To order additional copies of this book, contact:
Xlibris Corporation
1-888-795-4274
www.Xlibris.com
Orders@Xlibris.com
94333

Contents

Fasting

But seek first God's kingdom and his

righteousness, and all these things

will be given unto you.

—Matthew 6:33

Fasting

Purpose

· ·

The purpose of this book is to get Christians to understand how important it is to fast. We are disciples of Christ, and we need to perform as if we are.

> Then you will call upon me and come and pray to me, and i will listen to you. You will seek me and find me when you seek me with all your heart. I will be found by you, declares the Lord. (Jer 29:12-14a)

Key Verse

But seek first the kingdom of God and all his righteousness, and all these things will be added to your life. (Mt 6:33) Love, peace, joy, blessings, strength, houses, money, cars, food, and clothes.

Prayer

. . . .

Prayer is essential.

Spend time in conversation with God. Prayer is seeking God for someone or something. Prayer involves communion with God and recognition of his presence.

> And when you pray do not be like the hypocrites, for they love to pray, standing in the synagogues and on the street corners to be seen by men. I tell you the truth; they have received their reward in full. But when you pray, go into your room; close the door and pray to your father, who is unseen. Then your father, who sees what, is done in secret, will reward you. And when you pray, do not keep on babbling like pagans, for they think they will be heard because of their

many words. Do not be like them, for your father knows what you need before you ask him. (Mt 6:5-8)

Biblical Guidelines for Governing Prayer

We must have a great attitude for prayer and communion with God at all times.

Pray continually. (1 Thes 5:17)

In my prayers at all times; and I pray that at last by God's will the way may be opened for me to come to you. (Rom 1:10)

In the morning, O Lord you hear my voice; in the morning I lay my prayer before you and wait in expectation. (Ps 5:3)

But I call to God, and the Lord saves me. Evening, morning and noon I cry out in distress, and he hears my voice. (Ps 55:16, 17)

Spend Time Listening to God in Prayer

Let the morning bring me word of your unfailing love, for I have put my trust in you. Show me the way I should go. For to you I lift up my soul. (Ps 143:8)

Fasting

· ·

Fasting involves denying the body of natural foods and drinks, but it is also fasting from other things that we love and crave.

Fasting intensifies our sensitivity and opens us up to the Lord. Fasting is a time for placing the desires of the flesh under the control of the Holy Spirit. The soul needs to be chastened. Psalm 69:10 says, "When I wept, and chastened my soul with fasting. That was to my reproach." Or disgrace (meaning I saw things in myself that were not pleasing to God).

> When you fast, do not look somber as the hypocrites do, for they disfigure their faces to show men they are fasting. I tell you the truth; they have receive their reward in full. But when

you fast, put oil on your head and wash your face, so that it will not be obvious to men that you are fasting, but only to your father who is unseen; and your father, who sees what is done in secret, will reward you. (Mt 6:16-18)

The early church fasted, and we're to fast too.

Paul boasted about his sufferings when he fasted:

I have labored and toiled and have often gone without sleep, I have known hunger and thirst and have often gone without food. (2 Cor 11:27)

Fasting was also done corporately:

While they were worshiping the Lord and fasting, the Holy Spirit said, "Set apart for me Barnabas and Saul for the work to which I have called them." (Acts 13:2)

REV. CAROLYN YOUNG DAVIS

So when God calls on your life, you need to fast about it, or maybe God will give you a vision.

A fast will prepare you for whatever is coming in the future. Jesus was the greatest example of prayer and fasting. After fasting, the devil will come immediately to steal back the Word from you through sin, gossip, backbiting, and unforgivingness, so don't let the devil steal back what God has given you.

The Temptation of Jesus (Lk 4:1-13)

> Jesus full of the Holy Spirit, returned from the Jordan and was led by the spirit in the desert, where for forty days he was tempted by the devil. He ate nothing during those days, and at the end of them he was hungry. The devil said to him. "If you are the son of God, tell this stone to become bread."

Jesus answered, "It is written: man does not live on bread alone." [You have to talk to Satan, just like you have to talk to God.]

The devil led him up to a high place and showed him in an instant all the kingdoms of the world.

And he [Satan] said to him, "I will give you all their authority and splendor, for it has been given to me, and I can give it to anyone I want to.

"So, if you worship me, it will all be yours."

Jesus answered, "It is written: 'Worship the Lord your God and serve him only.'"

The devil led him [Jesus] to Jerusalem and had him stand on the highest point of the temple. "If you are the son of God," he [Satan] said "Throw yourself down from here.

For it is written 'He will command his angels concerning you to guard you carefully;

'They will lift you up in their hands so that you will not strike your foot against a stone.'"

Jesus answered, "It says: 'Do not put the Lord your God to the test.

When the devil had finished all this tempting, he left him [Jesus] until an opportune time.

I'm here to tell you that Satan will tempt you and return many times, so you must be ready for him, whether during a fast or just daily living.

God doesn't require us to fast forty days or even thirty days, but he does want us to fast sometimes.

We do not fast to lose weight, but we do lose weight when we fast. There is a race to be won before us, so let us run with patience. Food addiction is a sin. It is no better than alcohol. Most Christians are bound to the sin of food habits, and most of them don't know it. Angels will help break this yoke. Most Christians are wasting time and years (even when speaking in tongues). They are not fasting as they should. We should all fast like our Lord and Savior, Jesus Christ.

It Is Very Important to Receive What God Has to Offer

When the apostle in Jerusalem heard that Samaria had accepted the Word of God, they sent Peter and John to them. When they arrived, they prayed for them that they might receive the Holy Spirit.

—Acts 8:14, 15 NIV

Eternal Life

Healing

The Holy Spirit

All these are gifts, and there are many more if you want them. Just ask God for what you want and be specific and don't stop praying about it. The Word says to never cease to pray, meaning continue to pray always.

> And I will pray the father, and he shall give you another comforter, that he may abide with you forever; even the spirit of truth; whom the world cannot receive, because it seeth him not, neither knoweth him: but you know him; for he dwells with you, and shall be in you. (Jn 14:16, 17)

> Jesus often withdrew to lonely places and prayed. (Lk 5:16)

> One day Jesus was praying in a certain place when he finished, one of his disciples said to him Lord, teach us to pray, just as John taught his disciples. (Lk 11:1)

> In the early morning, while it was still dark, Jesus got up, left the house, and went away to a secluded place, and was praying there. (Mk 1:35)

REV. CAROLYN YOUNG DAVIS

What should be our attitudes in prayer and fasting:

We should have faith.

> And without faith it is impossible to please God, because anyone who comes to him must believe that he exists and that he rewards those who earnestly seek him. (Heb 11:6)

We should come humbled before the Lord.

> But as for me, when they were sick, my clothing was sackcloth: I humbled my soul with fasting: And my prayer returned into my own bosom. (Ps 35:13)

We should come desiring God's will for us.

> This is the confidence we have in approaching God: That if we ask anything according to his [will] he hears us and if we know that he hears

[us] whatever we [ask] we know that we have what we asked of him. (1 Jn 5:14,16)

Once we study the Word of God, we will know what his will is and we will only ask things of his will. We know he wants us blessed, he wants us healed, and he wants us delivered from the schemes of the Satan. Put on the whole armor of God.

Finally, be strong in the Lord and in the power of his might. Put on the whole armor of God, so that you will be able to stand against the strategies of the devil. For our struggle is not against flesh and blood, but against the rulers, against the power, against the world forces of this darkness, against the spiritual wickedness in the heavenly places. Therefore, take up the full armor of God. So that you will be able to resist in the evil day, and having done everything, to stand firm. Stand firm therefore, "Having girded your loins with truth. And having put on the breastplate of righteousness, having shod your feet with the preparation of the gospel of peace" In addition to all, taking up the shield of faith with which you will be able to extinguish all the flaming arrows of the evil one. "Take the helmet of salvation" and the sword of the spirit, which is the word of God. With all prayer and petition pray at all times in the spirit and with this in view, be on the alert with all perseverance and petition for all the saints. (Eph 6:10-18)

Obedience

For by Adam's disobedience we were made sinners, so by
obedience of Jesus we were made righteous (Rom 5:19). If
Jesus had to obey God, then who do we think we are? We
are no better than Jesus.

Confess these scriptures during your fasting.
"Have faith in God," Jesus answered. I tell you
the truth, if anyone says to this mountain, "Go,
throw yourself into the sea," and does not doubt
in his heart but believes that what he says will
happen, it will be done for him therefore I tell
you whatever you ask for in prayer, believe that
you have received it, and it will be yours and
when you stand praying, if you hold anything
against anyone, forgive him, so that your

father in heaven may forgive yours sins. (Mk 11:22-25)

We must be obedient to the Holy Spirit when we are fasting. We might have to be alone for a day to fast effectively. We can't hear the Holy Spirit speak to us when others are around us sometimes. If you don't recognize God's voice speaking to you, then read the Word of God and hear him through scriptures and prayer. The key to it all is obedience and love. The law of God is love.

Know to whom you obey. God's servants obey his voice through the Holy Spirit. We, as Christians, know the voice of God when we are filled with the Holy Spirit. If you are not filled, then ask God to fill you with the Holy Ghost. When we get saved, we are not filled with the Holy Spirit at that time.

Unless we ask at the time and even then the manifestation has to take place to let us know that we are filled by speaking in tongues. I don't mean the gift of tongues, but I mean the prayer language tongues. There is a difference.

We have the right to obey sin or righteousness unto death. You are a slave to the one you obey. We are the righteousness of God. Jesus died for that right. How could we not serve a God like that? A man who died for our sins so that we could have eternal life with him and the Father.

We must transform our minds (Rom 12:2). From disobedient to obedient first we must want to be obedient to the Holy Spirit. That's one step. The first step is to get saved by confessing Jesus Christ as your Lord and savior (Rom 10:9,10).

Say this prayer out loud and mean it from your heart:

> Dear Jesus, I repent for my sins and, Jesus, I
> believe you died on the cross for my sins and rose
> on the third day.

And, Jesus, come into my heart, be my Lord and savior, and fill me with the Holy Ghost and fire. Amen.

Now you are saved (born again), which means you are a Christian and heaven is your home. When you ask Jesus to come into your heart, that means he will rule and guide your life and you have given him that right. Jesus will not force you to do anything you don't want to do.

And he said: "I tell you the truth, unless you change and become like children, you will never enter the kingdom of heaven." (Mt 18:3)

You must decide whether you are going to be obedient to God and his spirit. You need to start reading scriptures at least fifteen minutes a day. Go to church on Sunday and find time for Sunday school and Bible study. All these will help you in your walk with God, and you will walk into the fast. If you don't have a Bible, then invest in a Bible. You need to buy an international version; it will break down scriptures for you.

All this is to prepare the new believer for fasting, and the present believer too.

Ask God for revelation and knowledge before you start reading your scriptures each day. Read Ephesians 1:17-23. Where the scripture says *our*, you say *my*; where it says *your*, you say *me*; and where it says *us*, you say *me*. God will give you revelation and knowledge of his scriptures over a period of time.

> I keep asking that the God of [my] Lord Jesus Christ, the glorious father, may give [me] the spirit of wisdom and revelation, so that [I] may know him better. I pray also that the eyes of [my] heart maybe enlightened in order that [I] may know the hope to which he has called [me], the riches of his glorious inheritance in the saints,

and his incomparably great power for [me] who believe[s]: That power is like the working of his mighty strength, which he exerted in Christ when he raised him from the dead and seated him at his right hand in the heavenly realms, far above all rule and authority, power and dominion and every title that can be given, not only in the present age but also in the one to come. And God placed all things under his feet and appointed him to be head over everything for the church, which is his body, the fullness of him who fills everything in every way? (Eph 1:17-23)

Once you get into the presence of God, you will begin to hear God speak to you. You are to spend some time alone with God. The mornings are the best times, but if you can't spend time in the morning then find time to spend with God. He loves you. He is the one who is going to make you beautiful—not only physically but also spiritually but you must obey. The Word of God will cleanse you, from bad eating habits to good eating habits.

Without faith in God it is impossible to please him (Heb 11:6).

The Holy Spirit inside you will tell you not to eat certain foods, and he will take the taste away from you if you ask him to. But remember, Satan will come to tempt you, and you must say, "No weapon formed against me shall prosper" (Is 54:17). I have given you power. I have given you power to tread on serpents and scorpions, and over all the power of the enemy: And nothing shall by any means hurt you.

In your prayer time each night, pray to God to take away the foods and drinks you know you should not have, and he will take those items away from you by the power of the Holy Ghost. After several days and nights, pray for the manifestation to come. God will answer your prayer. He just wants us to be sincere when we come to him for anything. He said in his Word, "If my Word abides in you and you abide in my Word, you can ask anything in my name, and it shall be done unto you."

Fasting

Fasting intensifies our sensitivity and opens us up to the Lord. Fasting is a time for placing the desires of the flesh under control of the Holy Spirit. The soul needs to be chastened (Ps 69:10). When I wept and chastened my soul with fasting, that was to my reproach or disgrace (meaning I saw things in myself that were not pleasing to God).

We should come with (self-) motivation (Ps 24:3, 4)

Who may ascend into the hill of the Lord?

Who may stand in his holy place?

He who has clean hands and a pure heart.

He who does not lift up his soul to an idol or swear by what is false.

Idols can be houses, cars, money, children, husbands and wives, and so on.

Make This Confession

I will be obedient to the voice of the Holy Ghost. I will fast and stop eating foods I should not eat. I have power within me to do what I set out to do.

> I can do all things through Christ which strengthen me. (Phil 4:13)

> Therefore if any man be in Christ, he is a new creature: Old things are passed away; behold, all things are become new. (2 Cor 5:17)

Keep in mind you are not the old person you used to be when you were not saved. You were a slave to the world, and now you are a slave to God. But that's a good thing because through this kind of slavery, you will receive the goodness of God.

But you are a chosen people, a royal priesthood, a holy nation, a people belonging to God, that you may declare the praise of him who called you out of darkness into his wonderful light. Now you are in the family of a royal priesthood. (1 Pt 2:9)

And we know that is the best family you can be in. You are the first and not the last. You are above and not beneath.

The First Day of Fasting

On the first day of fasting in the first week, you should fast only six hours a day if it's food that you are fasting from. If it's something like a certain food, then you can fast longer than six hours. If it is shopping or sexual immorality, then you can walk out of it by fasting. If it is smoking or drinking alcohol, you can walk out of it by fasting also.

If you are on medication, then you need to fast only a certain amount of hours each day for a week or two until you feel strength and you know it's from God. Only drink water, 100 percent juices, and natural fruits during the fast. You will feel hungry, but you must stand your ground and do all to stand. Don't eat any solid foods during the fast.

Fasting

Fasting enables us to become conductors of spiritual power for either blessing others or for bringing blessings to ourselves.

Fasting becomes prayer to the praying Christian. He humbles himself.

Fasting Intensifies the Power of Prayer

You must get spiritual food with each day of fasting. Take a day out of a week and fast for one month or every two months. There are several suggestions I would like to make for fasting: At 7:30 a.m. pray and praise God with songs. From 8:00 a.m. to 8:30 a.m. read scriptures. From 8:30 a.m. till 11:00 a.m. listen to the Word of God from tapes at home or in the car. It will heal your flesh and renew your mind;

it will clean out hearts and bitterness. From 11:00 a.m. till 1:00 p.m. you can drink 100 percent juice and water three times during the day. From 1:00 p.m. to 5:00 p.m. listen to the Word on tapes. Continue to praise and thank the Lord for his goodness and continue to listen to Christian music and meditate on the Word. Then take a nap from 5:00 p.m. to 7:00 p.m. From 7:00 p.m. to 10:00 p.m. watch Christian television. Then call it a night. If you have to work during the day of your fast, spend as much time as you can talking to God and listen to God talk back to you.

If you speak in an unknown tongue, then pray in the spirit (tongues) until you hear from God. He will speak back to you. If you don't speak in tongues, just keep praying in your language and you will hear from God.

Have a clear aim and be specific why you are fasting. Write it down.

You're preparing to diet after the fast. You're going to be dieting from foods you are used to eating, fasting for the

REV. CAROLYN YOUNG DAVIS

strength to keep dieting each day from the foods that put weight on you.

Fasting and prayer will bring about changes in your life.

> Because those who are led by the spirit of God are the sons of God. (Rom 8:14)

We must remember faith, faith in God then faith in ourselves.

> So faith comes by hearing, and hearing by the word of Christ. You must keep hearing and hearing the word of God. (Rom 10:17)

> Jesus said "If anyone is thirsty, let him come to me and drink. Whoever believes in me, as the scripture has said, streams of living water will flow from within him." By this he meant the spirit, whom those who believed in him were later to receive but at that time the spirit had not been

given, since Jesus had not yet been glorified. (Jn 7:37–39)

Conclusion

Prayer and fasting have answers to our lives, and most of all, love is the answer to our problems today. We must have faith in God as a believer. Every believer must practice love in order to get prayers answered, such as the abundant blessings.

We need a deeper relationship with the Father. Also, corporate prayer and fasting is vital and necessary for the church.

> But seek first his kingdom and his righteousness, and all these things will be given unto you [love, peace, joy, blessings, strength, healing, houses, cars, clothes, money, and so on]. (Mt 6:33)

May God bless you all.

Love you all.

Rev. C. Davis